The Definitive Cooking Book to Dash Diet Meals

Boost Metabolism and Get Healthy with this Selection of Fast and Cheap Recipes

Lola Rogers

Table of contents

Golden Eggplant Fries

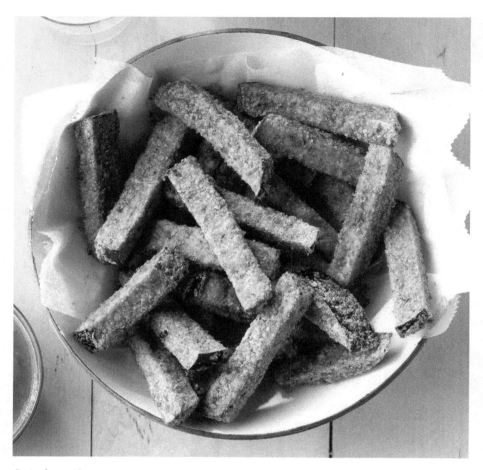

Serving: 8

Prep Time: 10 minutes

Cook Time: 15 minutes

Ingredients:

- 2 eggs
- 2 cups almond flour
- 2 tablespoons coconut oil, spray
- 2 eggplant, peeled and cut thinly
- Sunflower seeds and pepper

How To:

1. Preheat your oven to 400 degrees F.

2. Take a bowl and blend with sunflower seeds and black pepper.

3. Take another bowl and beat eggs until frothy.

4. Dip the eggplant pieces into the eggs.

5. Then coat them with the flour mixture.

6. Add another layer of flour and egg.

7. Then, take a baking sheet and grease with copra oil on top.

8. Bake for about quarter-hour .

9. Serve and enjoy!

Nutrition (Per Serving)

Calories: 212

Fat: 15.8g

Carbohydrates: 12.1g

Protein: 8.6g

Traditional Black Bean Chili

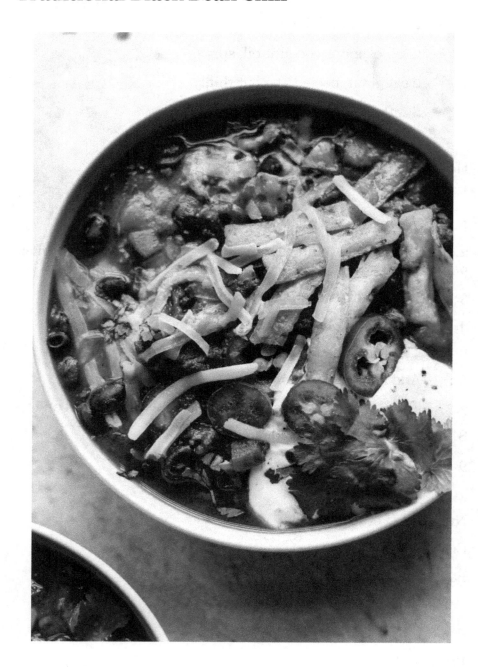

Serving: 4

Prep Time: 10 minutes

Cooking Time: 4 hours

Ingredients:

- 1 ½ cups red bell pepper, chopped
- 1 cup yellow onion, chopped
- 1 ½ cups mushrooms, sliced
- 1 tablespoon olive oil
- 1 tablespoon chili powder
- 2 garlic cloves, minced
- 1 teaspoon chipotle chili pepper, chopped
- ½ teaspoon cumin, ground
- 16 ounces canned black beans, drained and rinsed
- 2 tablespoons cilantro, chopped
- 1 cup tomatoes, chopped

How To:

1.   Add red bell peppers, onion, dill, mushrooms, flavor, garlic, chili pepper, cumin, black beans, tomatoes to your Slow Cooker.

2.   Stir well.

3. Place lid and cook on HIGH for 4 hours.

4. Sprinkle cilantro on top.

5. Serve and enjoy!

Nutrition (Per Serving)

Calories: 211

Fat: 3g

Carbohydrates: 22g

Protein: 5g

Very Wild Mushroom Pilaf

Serving: 4

Prep Time: 10 minutes

Cooking Time: 3 hours

Ingredients:

- 1 cup wild rice
- 2 garlic cloves, minced
- 6 green onions, chopped
- 2 tablespoons olive oil
- ½ pound baby Bella mushrooms
- 2 cups water

How To:

1.   Add rice, garlic, onion, oil, mushrooms and water to your Slow Cooker.

2.   Stir well until mixed.

3.   Place lid and cook on LOW for 3 hours.

4.   Stir pilaf and divide between serving platters.

5.   Enjoy!

Nutrition (Per Serving)

Calories: 210

Fat: 7g

Carbohydrates: 16g

Protein: 4g

Green Palak Paneer

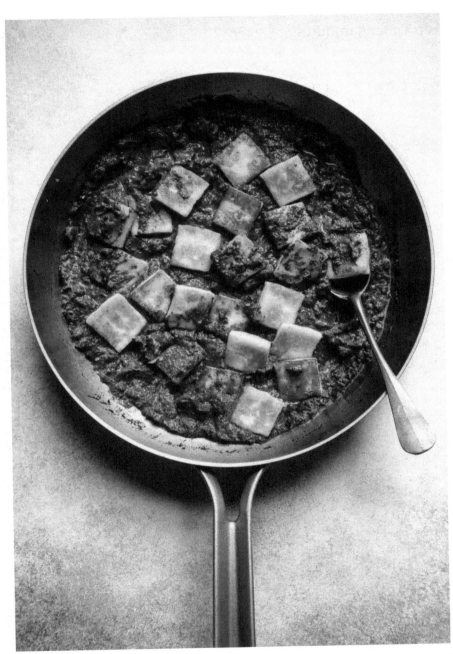

Serving: 4

Prep Time: 5 minutes

Cook Time: 10 minutes

Ingredients:

- 1-pound spinach
- 2 cups cubed paneer (vegan)
- 2 tablespoons coconut oil
- 1 teaspoon cumin
- 1 chopped up onion
- 1-2 teaspoons hot green chili minced up
- 1 teaspoon minced garlic
- 15 cashews
- 4 tablespoons almond milk
- 1 teaspoon Garam masala
- Flavored vinegar as needed

How To:

1.   Add cashews and milk to a blender and blend well.

2. Set your pot to Sauté mode and add coconut oil; allow the oil to heat up.

3. Add cumin seeds, garlic, green chilies, ginger and sauté for 1 minute.

4. Add onion and sauté for two minutes.

5. Add chopped spinach, flavored vinegar and a cup of water.

6. Lock up the lid and cook on high for 10 minutes.

7. Quick-release the pressure.

8. Add ½ cup of water and blend to a paste.

9. Add cashew paste, paneer and Garam Masala and stir thoroughly.

10. Serve over hot rice!

Nutrition (Per Serving)

Calories: 367

Fat: 26g

Carbohydrates: 21g

Protein: 16g

Pimento Cheese Sandwich

Ingredients

- Pimento cheese-Pasteurized process-2 oz-56.7 grams
- Multi-grain bread-Four slices regular-104 grams

Directions

1. Spread the pimento cheese over the bread.
2. Then, a slice of bread to form a sandwich. Enjoy!

Nutrition

Calories 488 Carbs 46g Fat 22g Protein 26g Fiber 8g Net carbs 38g Sodium 915mg Cholesterol 53mg

Coconut Oil Fat Bombs

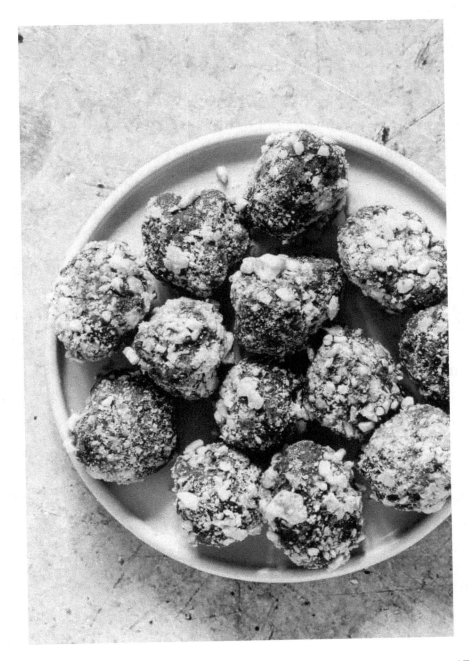

Ingredients

- Coconut oil-1 1/2 tbsp-20.8 grams
- Cocoa-Dry powder, unsweetened-3/4 tbsp-4.1 grams
- Honey-5/16 tsp-2 grams
- Salt-Table-1/8 tsp-0.57 grams

Directions

1.   Mix all the ingredients during a processor until the mixture is smooth and creamy.

2.   Pour into small-sized cube trays or silicone moulds and freeze.

3.   Once frozen, pop the copra oil fat bombs out of the pictures and store them during a freezer zip-top bag or jar. Enjoy!

Nutrition

Calories 194 Carbs 4g Fat 21g Protein 1g Fiber 2g Net carbs 3g Sodium 222mg Cholesterol 0mg

Apricot Jam and Almond Butter Sandwich

Ingredients

Multi-grain bread-Two slices regular-52 grams Jams and preserves-1 tbsp-20 grams

Almond butter-Nuts, every day, without salt, added-1 tbsp-16 grams

Directions

1.   Toast the bread optionally.

2.   Spread almond butter on one side and jam on the other side.

Nutrition

Calories 292 Carbs 39g Fat 11g Protein 10g Fiber 6g Net carbs 34g Sodium 206mg Cholesterol 0mg

Peanut Butter and Honey Toast

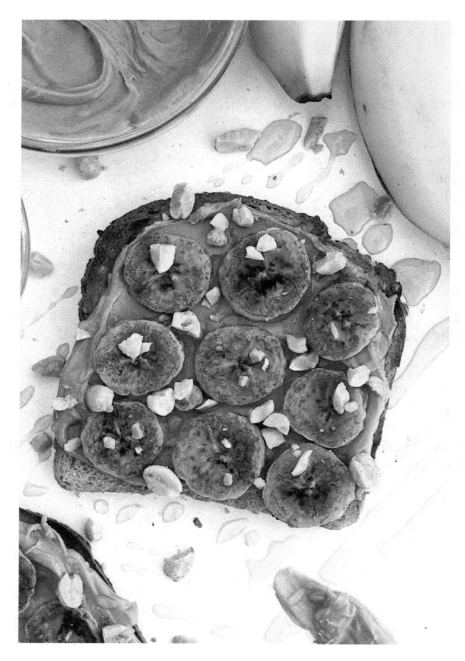

Ingredients

- Multi-grain bread-Two slices regular-52 grams
- Peanut butter-Smooth style, without salt-3 tbsp-48 grams
- Honey-2 tbsp-42 grams

Directions

1.   Toast the bread, and it is optionally.

2.   Spread peanut butter on the bread and sprinkle with honey. Enjoy!

Nutrition

Calories 553 Carbs 68g Fat 27g Protein 18g Fiber 6g Net carbs 62g Sodium 208mg

Cholesterol 0mg

Cucumber & Hummus

Ingredients

- Hummus-Commercial-1/4 cup-61.5 grams
- Cucumber-With peel, raw-1 cup slices-104 grams

Directions

Cut the cucumber into round slices and eat with hummus.

Nutrition

Calories 118

Carbs13g

Fat6g

Protein6g

Fiber4g

Net carbs8g

Carrot and Hummus Snack

Ingredients

Hummus-Commercial-2 tbsp-30 grams Baby carrots-Baby, raw-1 cup-246 grams

Directions

Dip carrots into hummus and enjoy!

Nutrition

Calories136Carbs25gFat3gProtein4gFiber9gNet

carbs16gSodium306mgCholesterol0mg

Cauliflower Bread Stick

Serving: 5 breadsticks

Prep Time: 10 minutes

Cooking Time: 48 minutes

Ingredients:

- 1 cup cashew cheese/ kite ricotta cheese
- 1 tablespoon organic almond butter
- 1 whole egg
- ½ teaspoon Italian seasoning
- ¼ teaspoon red pepper flakes
- 1/8 teaspoon kosher sunflower seeds
- 2 ups cauliflower rice, cooked for 3 minutes in microwave
- 3 teaspoons garlic, minced

- Parmesan cheese, grated

How To:

1.   Pre-heat your oven to 350 degrees F.

2.   Add almond butter during a small pan and melt over low heat

3.   Add red pepper flakes, garlic to the almond butter and cook for 2-3 minutes.

4.   Add garlic and almond butter mix to the bowl with cooked cauliflower and add the Italian seasoning.

5.   Season with sunflower seeds and blend , refrigerate for 10 minutes.

6.   Add cheese and eggs to the bowl and blend .

7.   Place a layer of parchment paper at rock bottom of a 9 x 9 baking dish and grease with cooking spray, add egg and mozzarella cheese mix to the cauliflower mix.

8.   Add mix to the pan and smooth to a skinny layer with the palms of your hand.

9.   Bake for half-hour , remove from oven and top with few shakes of parmesan and mozzarella.

10.   Cook for 8 minutes more.

11.   Enjoy!

Nutrition (Per Serving)

Total Carbs: 11.5g

Fiber: 2g

Protein: 10.7g

Fat: 20g

Bacon and Chicken Garlic Wrap

Serving: 4

Prep Time: 15 minutes

Cook Time: 10 minutes

Ingredients:

- 1 chicken fillet, cut into small cubes
- 8-9 thin slices bacon, cut to fit cubes
- 6 garlic cloves, minced

How To:

1. Pre-heat your oven to 400 degrees F.

2. Line a baking tray with aluminum foil .

3. Add minced garlic to a bowl and rub each chicken piece with it.

4. Wrap a bacon piece around each garlic chicken bite.

5. Secure with toothpick.

6.   Transfer bites to baking sheet, keeping a touch little bit of space between them.

7.   Bake for about 15-20 minutes until crispy.

8.   Serve and enjoy!

Nutrition (Per Serving)

Calories: 260

Fat: 19g

Carbohydrates: 5g

Protein: 22g

Chipotle Lettuce Chicken

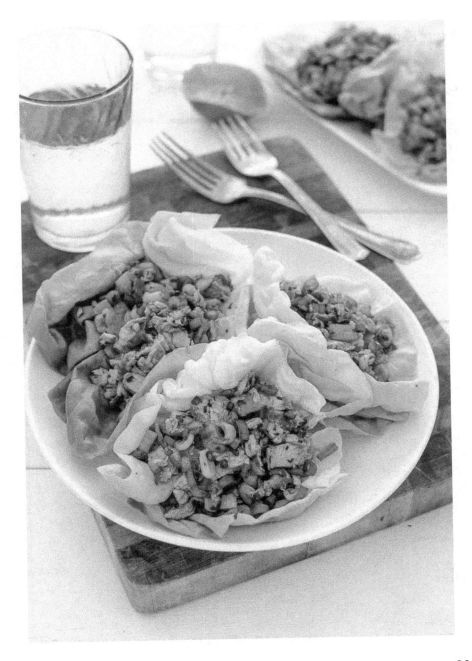

Serving: 6

Prep Time: 10 minutes

Cook Time: 25 minutes

Ingredients:

- 1-pound chicken breast, cut into strips
- Splash of olive oil
- 1 red onion, finely sliced
- 14 ounces tomatoes
- 1 teaspoon chipotle, chopped
- ½ teaspoon cumin
- Lettuce as needed
- Fresh coriander leaves
- Jalapeno chilies, sliced
- Fresh tomato slices for garnish
- Lime wedges

How To:

1.   Take a non-stick frypan and place it over medium heat.

2.   Add oil and warmth it up.

3.   Add chicken and cook until brown.

4.   Keep the chicken on the side.

5.   Add tomatoes, sugar, chipotle, cumin to an equivalent pan and simmer for 25 minutes until you've got a pleasant sauce.

6.   Add chicken into the sauce and cook for five minutes.

7.   Transfer the combination to a different place.

8.   Use lettuce wraps to require some of the mixture and serve with a squeeze of lemon.

9.   Enjoy!

Nutrition (Per Serving)

Calories: 332

Fat: 15g

Carbohydrates: 13g

Protein: 34g

Balsamic Chicken and Vegetables

Serving: 2

Prep Time: 15 minutes

Cook Time: 25 minutes

Ingredients:

- 4 chicken thigh, boneless and skinless
- 5 stalks of asparagus, halved
- 1 pepper, cut in chunks
- 1/2 red onion, diced
- ½ cup carrots, sliced
- 1 garlic cloves, minced
- 2-ounces mushrooms, diced
- ¼ cup balsamic vinegar
- 1 tablespoon olive oil
- ½ teaspoon stevia
- ½ tablespoon oregano
- Sunflower seeds and pepper as needed

How To:

1. Pre-heat your oven to 425 degrees F.

2. Take a bowl and add all of the vegetables and blend .

3. Add spices and oil and blend .

4. Dip the chicken pieces into spice mix and coat them well.

5. Place the veggies and chicken onto a pan during a single layer.

6. Cook for 25 minutes.

7. Serve and enjoy!

Nutrition (Per Serving)

Calories: 401

Fat: 17g

Net Carbohydrates: 11g

Protein: 48g

Cream Dredged Corn Platter

Serving: 3

Prep Time: 10 minutes

Cook Time: 4 hours

Ingredients:

- 3 cups corn
- 2 ounces cream cheese, cubed
- 2 tablespoons milk
- 2 tablespoons whipping cream
- 2 tablespoons butter, melted
- Salt and pepper as needed
- 1 tablespoon green onion, chopped

How To:

1.   Add corn, cheese , milk, light whipping cream , butter, salt and pepper to your Slow Cooker.

2.   provides it a pleasant toss to combine everything well.

3.   Place lid and cook on LOW for 4 hours.

4.   Divide the combination amongst serving platters.

5.   Serve and enjoy!

Nutrition (Per Serving)

Calories: 261

Fat: 11g

Carbohydrates: 17g

Protein: 6g

Chicken with Celery Root Puree

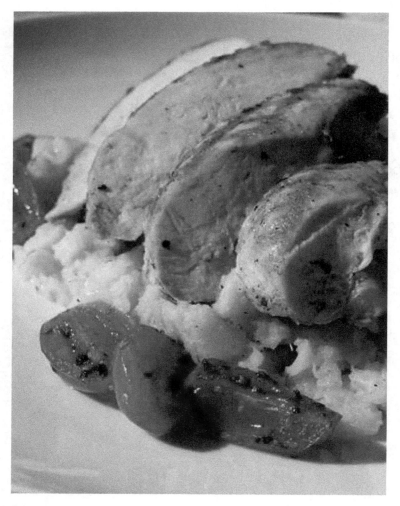

Ingredients

- Four boneless skinless chicken breast halves (6 ounces each)
- 1/2 teaspoon pepper

- 1/4 teaspoon salt

- Three teaspoons canola oil, divided

- One large celery root, peeled and chopped (about 3 cups)

- 2 cups diced peeled butternut squash

- One small onion, chopped

- Two garlic cloves, minced

- 2/3 cup unsweetened apple juice

Instructions

1. Sprinkle chicken with pepper and salt. Take an outsized skillet and coat with cooking spray, heat two teaspoons oil over medium heat. Brown chicken on each side . Remove chicken from pan.

2. Heat the remaining oil over medium-high within the same pan. Add celery root, squash and onion; cook and stir until squash is crisp-tender. Add garlic; cook 1 minute longer.

3. Return chicken to pan; add fruit juice . bring back a boil. Reduce heat; simmer, covered, 12-15 minutes or until a thermometer inserted in chicken reads 165°.

4. Remove chicken; keep warm. Cool vegetable mixture slightly. Process during a kitchen appliance until smooth. Return to pan and warmth through. Serve with chicken.

Nutrition Facts

328 calories, 8g fat (1g saturated fat), 94mg cholesterol, 348mg sodium, 28g carbohydrate (10g sugars, 5g fibre), 37g protein.

Apple-Cherry Pork Medallions

Ingredients

- One pork tenderloin (1 pound)
- One teaspoon minced fresh rosemary or 1/4 teaspoon dried rosemary, crushed
- One teaspoon minced fresh thyme or 1/4 teaspoon dried thyme
- 1/2 teaspoon celery salt
- One tablespoon olive oil
- One large apple, sliced
- 2/3 cup unsweetened apple juice
- Three tablespoons dried tart cherries
- One tablespoon honey
- One tablespoon cider vinegar
- One package (8.8 ounces) ready-to-serve brown rice

Instructions

1. Cut tenderloin crosswise into 12 slices; sprinkle with rosemary,

thyme and flavorer . during a huge skillet, heat oil over medium-excessive heat. Brown pork on both sides; do away with from pan.

2.   In the equal skillet, combine apple, fruit juice , cherries, honey and vinegar. Boil it and stirring to loosen browned bits

from pan. Reduce warmness; simmer, uncovered, 3-four minutes or simply till apple is tender.

3. Return meat to the pan, turning to coat with sauce; cook, covered, 3-4 minutes or till meat is tender. Meanwhile, put together rice keep with package deal directions; serve with meat mixture.

Nutrition Facts

349 calories, 9g fat (2g saturated fat), 64mg cholesterol, 179mg sodium, 37g carbohydrate (16g sugars, 4g fibre), and 25g protein.

Butternut Turkey Soup

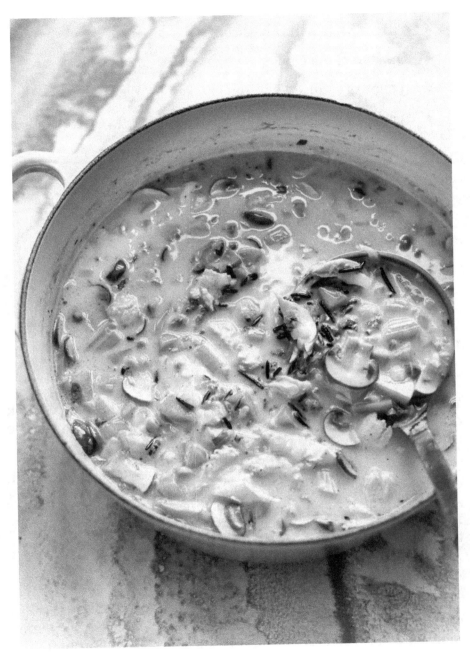

Ingredients

- Three shallots, thinly sliced
- One tsp of olive oil
- 3 cups of reduced-sodium chicken broth
- 3 cups of cubed peeled butternut squash (3/4-inch cubes)
- Two medium-sized red potatoes, cut into 1/2-inch cubes
- 1-1/2 cups of water
- Two teaspoons of minced fresh thyme
- 1/2 teaspoon pepper
- Two whole cloves
- 3 cups cubed cooked turkey breast

Instructions

1.	In a large-size saucepan coated with cooking spray, cook dinner shallots in oil over medium heat till tender. Stir within the broth, squash, potatoes, water, thyme and pepper.

2.	Place spices on a double thickness of cheesecloth; carry up corners of the material and tie with string to shape a bag. Stir into soup. bring back a boil. Reduce warmness; cowl and simmer for 10-15 mins or till vegetables are tender. Stir in turkey; warmth through. Discard spice bag.

Nutrition

192 calories, 2g fat (0 saturated fat), 60mg cholesterol, 332mg sodium, 20g carbohydrate (3g sugars, 3g fibre), 25g protein.

Black Bean & Sweet Potato Rice Bowls

Ingredients

- 3/4 cup uncooked long-grain rice
- 1/4 teaspoon garlic salt
- 1-1/2 cups water
- Three tablespoons olive oil, divided
- One large sweet potato, peeled and diced
- One medium red onion, finely chopped
- 4 cups chopped fresh kale (sturdy stems removed)
- One can (15 ounces) black beans, rinsed and drained
- Two tablespoons sweet chilli sauce
- Lime wedges, optional
- Additional sweet chilli sauce, optional

Instructions

1.   Place rice, flavorer and water during a large saucepan; bring back a boil. Reduce heat; simmer, covered until liquid is absorbed and rice is tender 15-20 minutes. Remove from heat; let stand 5 minutes.

2.   At an equivalent time take an outsized pan and warmth two tablespoons oil over medium-high heat; saute sweet potato 8 minutes. Add onion; cook and stir until potato is tender 4-6 minutes. Add kale; cook and stir until tender, 3-5 minutes. Stir in beans; heat through.

3.   Gently stir two tablespoons chilli sauce and remaining oil into rice; increase potato mixture. If you would like , serve with lime wedges and extra chilli sauce.

Nutrition

435 calories, 11g fat (2g saturated fat), 0 cholesterol, 405mg sodium, 74g carbohydrate (15g sugars, 8g fibre), 10g protein.

Pepper Ricotta Primavera

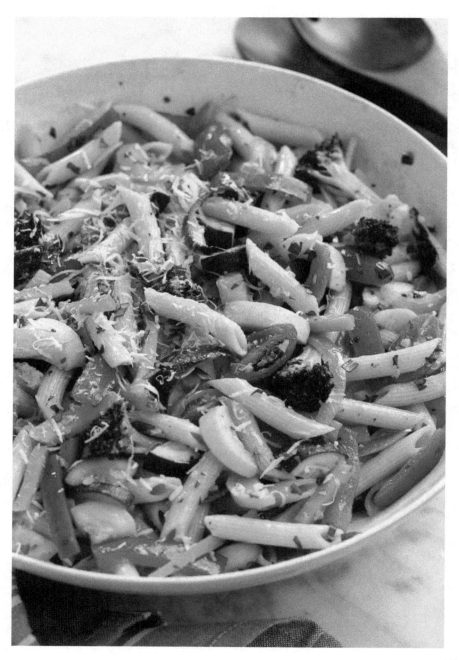

Ingredients

- 1 cup part-skim ricotta cheese
- 1/2 cup fat-free milk
- Four teaspoons olive oil
- One garlic clove, minced
- 1/2 teaspoon crushed red pepper flakes
- One medium green pepper, julienned
- One medium sweet red pepper, julienned
- One medium fresh yellow pepper, julienned
- One medium zucchini, sliced 1 cup frozen peas, thawed
- 1/4 teaspoon dried oregano
- 1/4 teaspoon dried basil
- 6 ounces fettuccine, cooked and drained

Instructions

1.   Whisk together ricotta cheese and milk; put aside . Take an outsized skillet, heat oil over medium heat. Add garlic and pepper; saute 1 minute. Add subsequent seven ingredients. Cook and blend over medium heat until vegetables are crisptender, about 5 minutes.

2.   Add cheese mixture to fettuccine; top with vegetables. Toss to coat. Serve immediately.

Nutrition

229 calories, 7g fat (3g saturated fat), 13mg cholesterol, 88mg sodium, 31g carbohydrate (6g sugars, 4g fibre), 11g protein.

Butternut and Garlic Soup

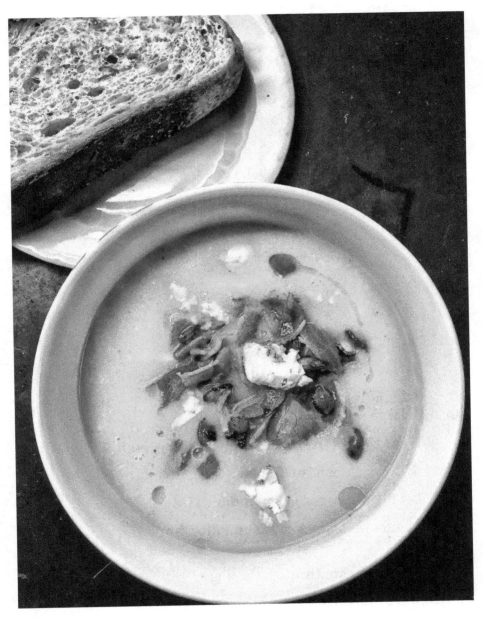

Serving: 4

Prep Time: 5 minutes

Cook Time: 35 minutes

Ingredients:

- 4 cups butternut squash, cubed
- 4 cups vegetable broth, stock
- ½ cup low fat cream
- 2 garlic cloves, chopped
- Pepper to taste

How To:

1. Add butternut squash, garlic cloves, broth, salt and pepper during a large pot.

2. Place the pot over medium heat and canopy with the lid.

3. Bring back boil then reduce the temperature.

4. Let it simmer for 30-35 minutes.[MOU7]

5. Blend the soup for 1-2 minutes until you get a smooth mixture.

6. Stir the cream through the soup.

7. Serve and enjoy!

Nutrition (Per Serving)

Calories: 180

Fat: 14g

Carbohydrates: 21g

Protein: 3g

Minty Avocado Soup

Serving: 4

Prep Time: 10 minutes + Chill time

Cook Time: nil

Ingredients:

- 1 avocado, ripe
- 1 cup coconut almond milk, chilled
- 2 romaine lettuce leaves
- 20 mint leaves, fresh
- 1 tablespoon lime juice
- Sunflower seeds, to taste

How To:

1. Activate your slow cooker and add all the ingredients into it.
2. Mix them during a kitchen appliance .
3. Make a smooth mixture.
4. Let it chill for 10 minutes.
5. Serve and enjoy!

Nutrition (Per Serving)

Calories: 280

Fat: 26g

Carbohydrates: 12g

Protein: 4g

Celery, Cucumber and Zucchini Soup

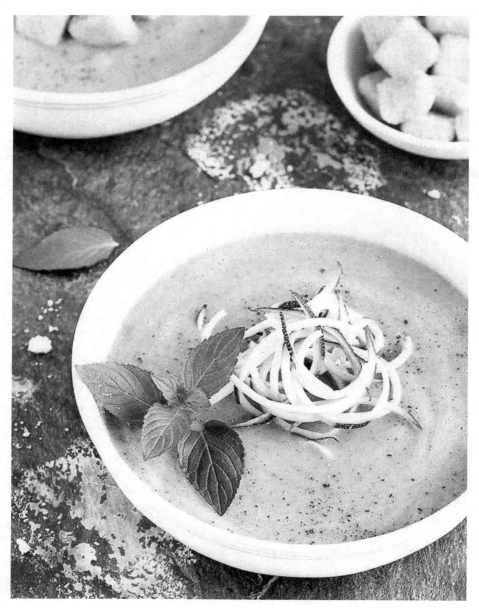

Serving: 2

Prep Time: 10 minutes + Chill time

Cook Time: nil

Ingredients:

- 3 celery stalks, chopped
- 7 ounces cucumber, cubed
- 1 tablespoon olive oil
- 2/5 cup fresh cream, 30%, low fat
- 1 red bell pepper, chopped
- 1 tablespoon dill, chopped
- 10 ½ ounces zucchini, cubed
- Sunflower seeds and pepper, to taste

How To:

1. Put the vegetables during a juicer and juice.
2. Then mix within the vegetable oil and fresh cream.
3. Season with sauce and pepper.
4. Garnish with dill.
5. Serve it chilled and enjoy!

Nutrition (Per Serving)

Calories: 325

Fat: 32g

Carbohydrates: 10g

Protein: 4g

Rosemary and Thyme Cucumber Soup

Serving: 3

Prep Time: 10 minutes + Chill time

Cook Time: nil

Ingredients:

- 4 cups vegetable broth
- 1 teaspoon thyme, freshly chopped
- 1 teaspoon rosemary, freshly chopped
- 2 cucumbers, sliced1 cup low fat cream
- 1 pinch of sunflower seeds

How To:

1. Take an outsized bowl and add all the ingredients.
2. Whisk well.
3. Blend until smooth by using an immersion blender.
4. Let it chill for 1 hour.
5. Serve and enjoy!

Nutrition (Per Serving)

Calories: 111

Fat: 8g

Carbohydrates: 4g

Protein: 5g

Guacamole Soup

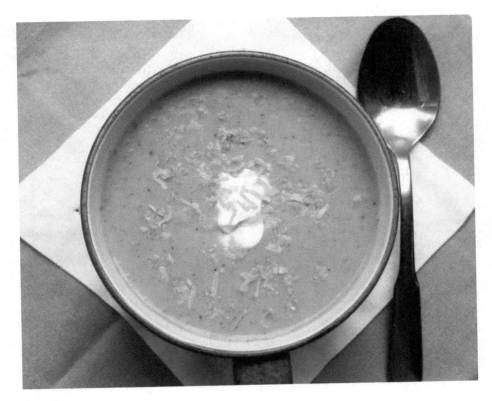

Serving: 3

Prep Time: 10 minute + Chill time

Cook Time: nil

Ingredients:

- 3 cups vegetable broth 2 ripe avocados, pitted

- ½ cup cilantro, freshly chopped
- 1 tomato, chopped
- ½ cup low fat cream
- Sunflower seeds & black pepper, to taste

How To:

1. Add all the ingredients into a blender.
2. Blend until creamy by using an immersion blender.
3. Let it chill for 1 hour.
4. Serve and enjoy!

Nutrition (Per Serving)

Calories: 289

Fat: 26g

Carbohydrates: 5g

Protein: 10g

Chickpea Salad

Serving: 4

Prep Time: 6 minutes

Cook Time: Nil

Ingredients:

- 1 cup canned chickpeas, drained and rinsed.
- 2 spring onions, thinly sliced.
- 1 small cucumber, diced.
- 2 green bell peppers, chopped.
- 2 tomatoes, diced.
- 2 tablespoons fresh parsley, chopped.
- 1 teaspoon capers, drained and rinsed.
- Half a lemon, juiced.
- 2 tablespoons sunflower oil.
- 1 tablespoon red wine vinegar.
- Pinch of dried oregano.
- Sunflower seeds and pepper to taste

How To:

1.   Take a medium sized bowl and add chickpeas, spring onions, cucumber, bell pepper, tomato, parsley and capers.

2.   Take another bowl and mix in the rest of the ingredients, pour mixture over chickpea salad and toss well.

3.   Coat and serve, enjoy!

Nutrition (Per Serving)

Calories: 74

Fat: 0.7g

Carbohydrates: 16g

Protein: 2g

Dashing Bok Choy Samba

Serving: 3

Prep Time: 5 minutes

Cook Time: 15 minutes

Ingredients:

- 4 bok choy, sliced
- 1 onion, sliced
- ½ cup Parmesan cheese, grated
- 4 teaspoons coconut cream
- Sunflower seeds and freshly ground black pepper, to taste

How To:

1. Mix bok choy with black pepper and sunflower seeds.
2. Take a cooking pan, heat the oil and to sauté sliced onion for 5 minutes.
3. Then add cream and seasoned bok choy.
4. Cook for 6 minutes.
5. Stir in Parmesan cheese and cover with a lid.

6. Reduce the heat to low and cook for 3 minutes.

7. Serve warm and enjoy!

Nutrition (Per Serving)

Calories: 112

Fat: 4.9g

Carbohydrates: 1.9g

Protein: 3g

Simple Avocado Caprese Salad

Serving: 6

Prep Time: 15 minutes

Cook Time: 29 minutes

Ingredients:

- 2 avocados, cubed
- 1 cup cherry tomatoes, halved
- 8 ounces mozzarella balls, halved
- 2 tablespoons finely chopped fresh basil
- 2 tablespoons olive oil
- 2 tablespoons balsamic vinegar
- 1 tablespoon sunflower seeds
- Fresh ground black pepper

How To:

1. Take a bowl and add the listed ingredients, toss them well until

thoroughly mixed.

2.   Season with pepper according to your taste.

3.   Serve and enjoy!

Nutrition (Per Serving)

Calories: 358

Fat: 30g

Carbohydrates: 9g

Protein: 14g

The Rutabaga Wedge Dish

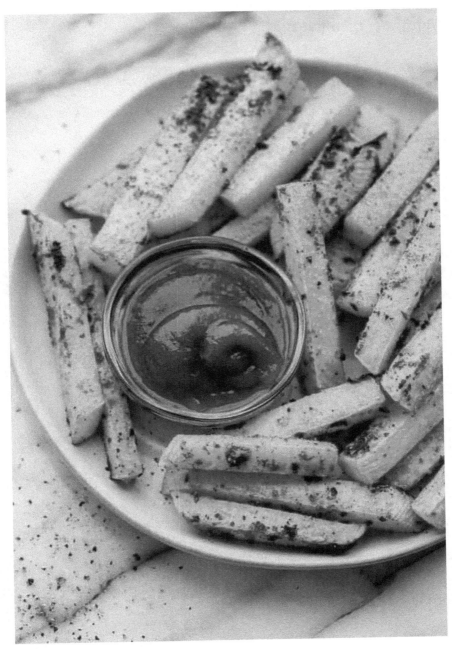

Serving: 4

Prep Time: 15 minutes

Cook Time: 45 minutes

Ingredients:

- 2 medium rutabagas, medium, cleaned and peeled
- 4 tablespoons almond butter
- ½ teaspoon sunflower seeds
- ½ teaspoon onion powder
- 1/8 teaspoon black pepper
- ½ cup buffalo wing sauce
- ¼ cup blue cheese dressing, low fat and low sodium
- 2 green onions, chopped

How To:

1. Pre-heat your oven to 400 degrees F.

2. Line a baking sheet with parchment paper.

3. Wash and peel rutabagas, clean and peel them, and cut into wedge shapes.

4.   Take a skillet and place it over low heat, add almond butter and melt.

5.   Stir in onion powder, sunflower seeds, onion, black pepper.

6.   Use seasoned almond butter to coat wedges.

7.   Arrange wedges in a single layer on the baking sheet.

8.   Bake for 30 minutes.

9.   Remove and coat in buffalo sauce and return to oven.

10.   Bake for 15 minutes more.

11.   Place wedges on serving plate and trickle with blue cheese dressing.

12.   Garnish with chopped green onion and enjoy!

Nutrition (Per Serving)

Calories: 235

Fat: 15g

Carbohydrates: 10g

Protein: 2.5g

Red Coleslaw

Serving: 4

Prep Time: 10 minutes

Cook Time: 0 minutes

Ingredients:

- 1 2/3 pounds red cabbage
- 2 tablespoons ground caraway seeds
- 1 tablespoon whole grain mustard
- 1 1/4 cups mayonnaise
- Sunflower seeds and black pepper

How To:

1. Take a large bowl and all the remaining ingredients.
2. Mix it well and let it sit for 10 minutes.
3. Serve and enjoy!

Nutrition (Per Serving)

Calories: 406

Fat: 40.8g

Carbohydrates: 10g

Protein: 2.2g

Spanish Mussels

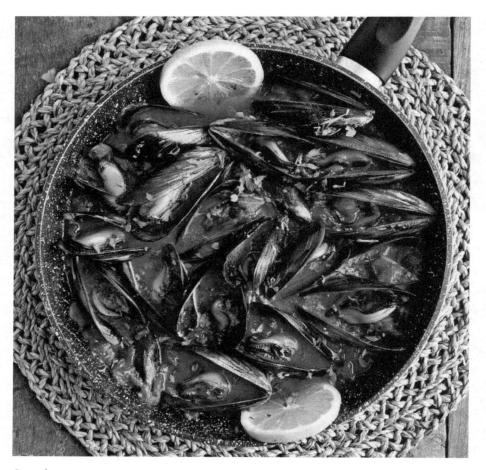

Serving: 4

Prep Time: 10 minutes

Cook Time: 23 minutes

Ingredients:

- tablespoons olive oil
- pounds mussels, scrubbed
- Pepper to taste
- cups canned tomatoes, crushed
- shallot, chopped
- garlic cloves, minced
- cups low sodium vegetable stock
- 1/3 cup cilantro, chopped

How To:

1. Take a pan and place it over medium-high heat, add shallot and stir-cook for 3 minutes.

2. Add garlic, stock, tomatoes, pepper, stir and reduce heat, simmer for 10 minutes.

3. Add mussels, cilantro, and toss.

4. Cover and cook for 10 minutes more.

5. Serve and enjoy!

Nutrition (Per Serving)

Calories: 210

Fat: 2g

Carbohydrates: 5g

Protein: 8g

Tilapia Broccoli Platter

Serving: 2

Prep Time: 4 minutes

Cook Time: 14 minutes

Ingredients:

- Ounce tilapia, frozen
- 1 tablespoon almond butter
- 1 tablespoon garlic, minced
- 1 teaspoon lemon pepper seasoning
- 1 cup broccoli florets, fresh

How To:

1. Pre-heat your oven to 350 degrees F.
2. Add fish in aluminum foil packets.
3. Arrange broccoli around fish.
4. Sprinkle lemon pepper on top.
5. Close the packets and seal.
6. Bake for 14 minutes.

7.   Take a bowl and add garlic and almond butter, mix well and keep the mixture on the side.

8.   Remove the packet from oven and transfer to platter.

9.   Place almond butter on top of the fish and broccoli, serve and enjoy!

Nutrition (Per Serving)

Calories: 362

Fat: 25g

Carbohydrates: 2g

Protein: 29g

Salmon with Peas and Parsley Dressing

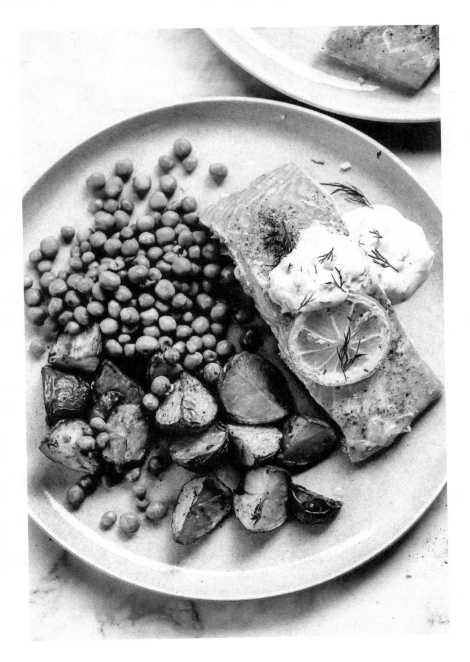

Serving: 4

Prep Time: 15 minutes

Cook Time: 15 minutes

Ingredients:

- 16 ounces salmon fillets, boneless and skin-on
- 1 tablespoon parsley, chopped
- 10 ounces peas
- 9 ounces vegetable stock, low sodium
- 2 cups water
- ½ teaspoon oregano, dried
- ½ teaspoon sweet paprika
- 2 garlic cloves, minced
- A pinch of black pepper

How To:

1. Add garlic, parsley, paprika, oregano and stock to a kitchen appliance and blend.

2. Add water to your Instant Pot.

3. Add steam basket.

4.   Add fish fillets inside the steamer basket.

5.   Season with pepper.

6.   Lock the lid and cook on high for 10 minutes.

7.   Release the pressure naturally over 10 minutes .

8.   Divide the fish amongst plates.

9.   Add peas to the steamer basket and lock the lid again, cook on high for five minutes.

10.   Quick release the pressure.

11.   Divide the peas next to your fillets and serve with the parsley dressing drizzled

12.   on top

13.   Enjoy!

Nutrition (Per Serving)

Calories: 315

Fat: 5g

Carbohydrates: 14g

Protein: 16g

Mackerel and Orange Medley

Serving: 4

Prep Time: 10 minutes

Cook Time: 10 minutes

Ingredients:

- mackerel fillets, skinless and boneless
- spring onion, chopped
- 1 teaspoon olive oil
- 1-inch ginger piece, grated
- Black pepper as needed
- Juice and zest of 1 whole orange
- 1 cup low sodium fish stock

How To:

1.   Season the fillets with black pepper and rub vegetable oil .

2.   Add stock, fruit juice , ginger, orange peel and onion to Instant Pot.

3.   Place a steamer basket and add the fillets.

4.   Lock the lid and cook on high for 10 minutes.

5.   Release the pressure naturally over 10 minutes.

6.   Divide the fillets amongst plates and drizzle the orange sauce from the pot over the fish.

7.   Enjoy!

Nutrition (Per Serving)

Calories: 200

Fat: 4g

Carbohydrates: 19g

Protein: 14g

Spicy Chili Salmon

Serving: 4

Prep Time: 10 minutes

Cook Time: 7 minutes

Ingredients:

- salmon fillets, boneless and skin-on
- 2 tablespoons assorted chili peppers, chopped
- Juice of 1 lemon
- 1 lemon, sliced
- 1 cup water
- Black pepper

How To:

1.   Add water to the moment Pot.

2.   Add steamer basket and add salmon fillets, season the fillets with salt and pepper.

3.   Drizzle juice on top.

4.   Top with lemon slices.

5.   Lock the lid and cook on high for 7 minutes.

6.   Release the pressure naturally over 10 minutes.

7.   Divide the salmon and lemon slices between serving plates.

8.   Enjoy!

Nutrition (Per Serving)

Calories: 281

Fats: 8g

Carbs: 19g

Protein:7g

Panko-Crusted Cod

Prep time: 10 minutes

Cook time: 15 minutes

Servings: 2

Ingredients

- Panko-style breadcrumbs – ¼ cup
- Garlic - 1 clove, minced
- Extra-virgin olive oil – 1 Tbsp.
- Nonfat Greek yogurt – 3
- Tbsp. Mayonnaise – 1 Tbsp.
- Lemon juice – 1 ½ tsp.
- Tarragon – ½ tsp.
- Pinch of salt
- Cod – 10 ounces, cut into two portions

Method

1. Preheat the oven to 425F.
2. Coat a baking pan with cooking spray.

3. In a bowl, combine olive oil, garlic, and breadcrumbs.

4. In another bowl, combine lemon juice, mayonnaise, yogurt, tarragon, and salt.

5. Place fish in the baking pan. Top each piece with one-half yogurt mixture then 1/3 breadcrumb mixture.

6. Bake in the oven for 15 minutes.

7. Serve.

Nutritional Facts Per Serving

Calories: 225

Fat: 10g

Carb: 13g

Protein: 18g

Sodium 270mg

Grilled Salmon And Asparagus With Lemon Butter

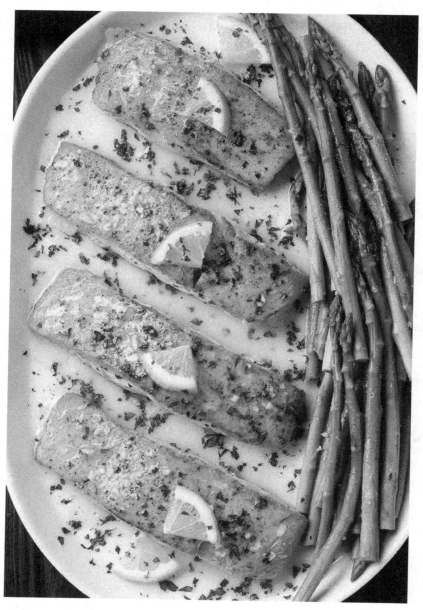

Prep time: 10 minutes

Cook time: 20 minutes

Servings: 4

Ingredients

- Salmon – 1 ¼ pound, cut into 4 portions
- Asparagus – 2 bunches, ends trimmed
- Olive oil cooking spray
- Salt – ½ tsp.
- Freshly ground black pepper – ¼ tsp.
- Garlic powder – ¼ tsp.
- Olive oil – 1 Tbsp.
- Butter – 1 Tbsp.
- Lemon juice – 3 Tbsp.

Method

1.	On a baking sheet, place the salmon and asparagus. Spray lightly with cooking spray. Season with salt, pepper, and garlic powder.

2.	Grease and preheat grill. Place salmon and asparagus on it.

3.	Grill total 6 minutes, 3 mintues per side, or until opaque, turning once.

4. Grill the asparagus for 5 to 7 minutes, or until tender, turning occasionally.

5. In a bowl, place butter, olive oil, and lemon juice. Microwave to melt.

6. Drizzle fish with this mixture.

7. Serve.

Nutritional Facts Per Serving

Calories: 190

Fat: 8g

Carb: 6g

Protein: 24g

Sodium 445mg

Pan-Roasted Fish Fillets With Herb Butter

Prep time: 10 minutes

Cook time: 5 minutes

Servings: 2

Ingredients

- Fish fillets – 2 (5-ounce each) ½ to 1 inch thick
- Salt – ¼ tsp.
- Ground black pepper
- Olive oil – 3 Tbsp.
- Unsalted butter -1 Tbsp. divided
- Fresh thyme – 2 sprigs
- Chopped flat-leaf parsley - 1 Tbsp.
- Lemon wedges

Method

1. Rub the fish with pepper and salt.
2. Heat oil in a skillet.

3. Place fillets and cook until around the edges, about 2 to 3 minutes. Then flip the fillets and add the butter and thyme to the pan.

4. Baste the fish with melted butter until golden all over, about 2 minutes.

5. Serve with chopped parsley and lemon wedges.

Nutritional Facts Per Serving

Calories: 369

Fat: 26.9g

Carb: 1g

Protein: 30.5g

Sodium 62mg

Chili Macadamia Crusted Tilapia

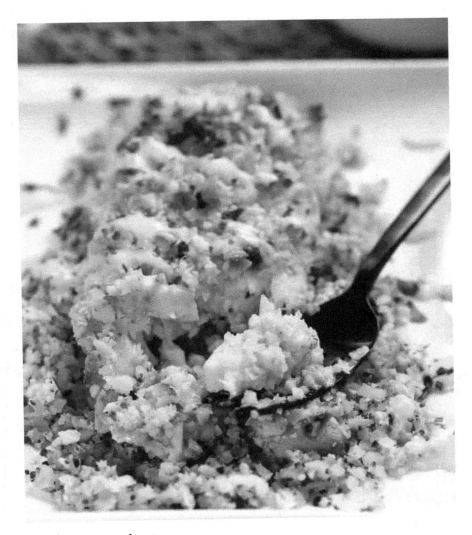

Prep time: 20 minutes

Cook time: 7 minutes

Servings: 4

Ingredients

- Tilapia fillets – 4
- Macadamia nuts – ½ cup, chopped coarsely
- Whole wheat panko crumbs – ½ cup
- Chili powder – 1 tsp.
- Cayenne pepper – ¼ tsp.
- Paprika – ¼ tsp.
- Salt – ¼ tsp.
- Pepper – ¼ tsp.
- Egg – 1
- Olive oil – 3 Tbsp.

Method

1. In a bowl, combine panko crumbs, nuts, chili powder, cayenne pepper, paprika, salt, and pepper.

2. Whisk egg in another bowl and set aside.

3. Heat the olive oil in a skillet.

4. Dredge each tilapia fillet in the egg and then coat it in the macadamia-spice-panko mixture.

5. Cook fillets until browned and cooked through, about 3 minutes on each side.

6.   Serve.

Nutritional Facts Per Serving

Calories: 351

Fat: 26.5g

Carb: 5.7g

Protein: 25.7g

Sodium 234mg

Broiled White Sea Bass

Prep time: 5 minutes

Cook time: 10 minutes

Servings: 2

Ingredients

- White sea bass fillets – 2, each 4 ounces
- Lemon juice – 1 Tbsp.
- Garlic – 1 tsp. minced
- Salt-free herb seasoning blend – ¼ tsp.
- Ground black pepper to taste

Method

1.   Heat the broiler (grill).

2.   Place the rack very close (4 inches) to the heat source.

3.   Place the fillets in a greased baking pan.

4.   Sprinkle the fillets with herbed seasoning, garlic, lemon juice, and pepper.

5.   Broil (grill) until opaque throughout, about 8 to 10 minutes

6.   Serve.

Nutritional Facts Per Serving

Calories: 102

Fat: 2g

Carb: 1g

Protein: 21g

Sodium 77mg

Beef With Pea Pods

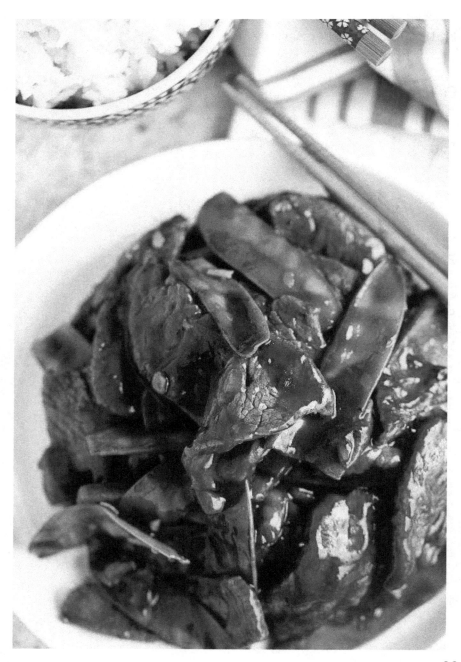

Prep time: 5 minutes

Cook time: 10 minutes

Servings: 4

Ingredients

- Thin beef steak – ¾ pound, sliced into thin strips
- Peanut oil – 1 Tbsp.
- Scallions – 3, sliced
- Garlic – 2 cloves, minced
- Minced fresh ginger – 2 tsp.
- Fresh pea pods – 4 cups, trimmed
- Homemade soy sauce – 3 Tbsp.
- Cooked brown rice – 4 cups

Method

1. Heat the oil in a pan.
2. Add the garlic, scallions, and ginger.
3. Stir-fry for 30 seconds.
4. Add the sliced beef and stir-fry for 5 minutes, or until beef has browned.

5.   Add pea pods and soy sauce and stir-fry for 3 minutes.

6.   Remove from heat.

7.   Serve with rice.

Homemade soy sauce

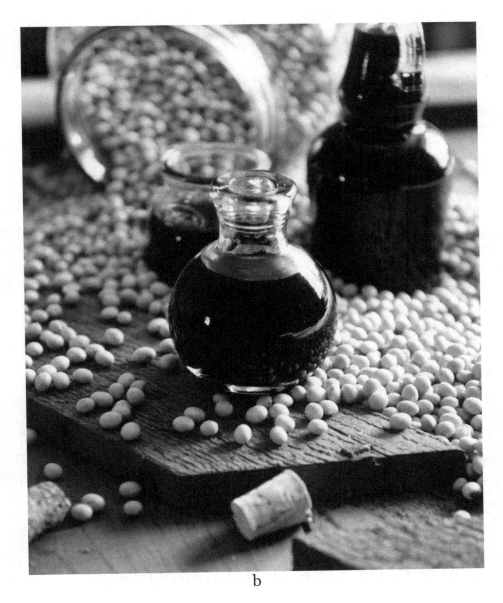

b

- Molasses – ¼ cup
- Unflavored rice wine vinegar – 3 Tbsp.

- Water – 1 Tbsp.
- Sodium-free beef bouillon granules – 1 tsp.
- Freshly ground black pepper - ½ tsp.

Method

1.   Mix everything in a saucepan and heat on low for 1 minute.
2.   Serve.

Nutritional Facts Per Serving

Calories: 466

Fat: 11g

Carb: 64g

Protein: 27g

Sodium 71mg

Whole-Grain Rotini With Ground Pork

Prep time: 10 minutes

Cook time: 25 minutes

Servings: 6

Ingredients

- Whole-grain rotini - 1 (13-ounce) package
- Lean ground pork – 1 pound
- Red onion – 1, chopped
- Garlic – 3 cloves, minced
- Bell pepper – 1, chopped
- Pumpkin puree – 1 cup
- Ground sage – 2 tsp.
- Ground rosemary – 1 tsp.
- Ground black pepper to taste

Method

1.   Cook the pasta (follow the package insturctions). Omit salt, drain and set aside.

2.   Heat a pan over medium heat. Add onion, garlic, and ground pork and sauté for 2 minutes.

3.   Add bell pepper and sauté for 5 minutes.

4.   Remove from heat. Add pasta to the pan along with remaining ingredients.

5.   Mix and serve.

Nutritional Facts Per Serving

Calories: 331

Fat: 7g

Carb: 45g

Protein: 23g

Sodium 48mg

Roasted Pork Loin With Herbs

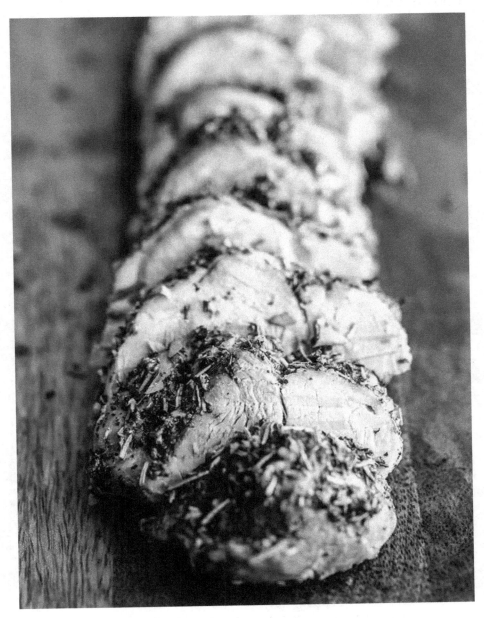

Prep time: 20 minutes

Cook time: 1 hour

Servings: 4

Ingredients

- Boneless pork loin roast – 2 lbs.
- Garlic – 3 cloves, minced
- Dried rosemary – 1 Tbsp.
- Dried thyme – 1 tsp.
- Dried basil – 1 tsp.
- Salt – ¼ tsp.
- Olive oil – ¼ cup
- White wine – ½ cup
- Pepper to taste

Method

1.   Preheat the oven to 350F.

2.   Crush the garlic with thyme, rosemary, basil, salt, and pepper, making a paste. Set aside.

3.   Use a knife to pierce meat several times.

4. Press the garlic paste into the slits.

5. Rub the meat with the rest of the garlic mixture and olive oil.

6. Place pork loin into the oven, turning and basting with pan liquids, until the pork reaches 145F, about 1 hour. Remove the pork from the oven.

7. Place the pan over heat and add white wine, stirring the brown bits on the bottom.

8. Top roast with sauce.

9. Serve.

Nutritional Facts Per Serving

Calories: 464

Fat: 20.7g

Carb: 2.4g

Protein: 59.6g

Sodium 279mg

Garlic Lime Pork Chops

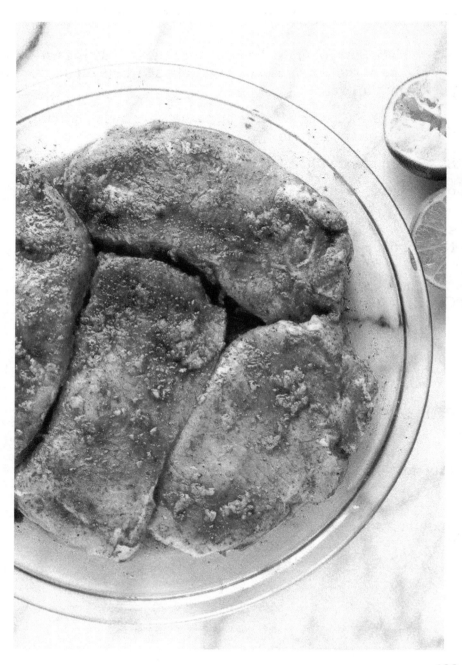

Prep time: 20 minutes

Cook time: 10 minutes

Servings: 4

Ingredients

- Lean boneless pork chops – 4 (6-oz. each)
- Garlic – 4 cloves, crushed
- Cumin – ½ tsp.
- Chili powder - ½ tsp.
- Paprika - ½ tsp.
- Juice of ½ lime
- Lime zest – 1 tsp.
- Kosher salt - ¼ tsp.
- Fresh pepper to taste

Method

1. In a bowl, season pork with cumin, chili powder, paprika, garlic salt, and pepper. Add lime juice and zest.

2. Marinate the pork for 20 minutes.

3. Line a broiler pan with foil.

4.   Place the pork chops on the broiler pan and broil for 5 minutes on each side or until browned.

5.   Serve.

Nutritional Facts Per Serving

Calories: 233

Fat: 13.2g

Carb: 4.3g

Protein: 25.5g

Sodium 592mg